7/11 cer

EPIDEMICS AND SOCIETY ™

EBOLA

AUBREY STIMOLA

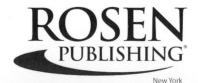

ROSEN
PUBLISHING®

New York

For my husband, Peter, who sees nothing but silver linings

Published in 2011 by The Rosen Publishing Group, Inc.
29 East 21st Street, New York, NY 10010

First Edition

Library of Congress Cataloging-in-Publication Data

Stimola, Aubrey.
Ebola / Aubrey Stimola.—1st ed.
    p. cm.—(Epidemics and society)
Includes bibliographical references and index.
ISBN 978-1-4358-9433-4 (lib. bdg.)
1. Ebola virus disease—Popular works. I. Title.
RC140.5.S75 2011
614.5'7—dc22

                                                          2009043451

Manufactured in the United States of America

CPSIA Compliance Information: Batch #S10YA: For further information, contact Rosen Publishing, New York, New York, at 1-800-237-9932.

On the cover: An image of the Ebola virus.

CONTENTS

INTRODUCTION **4**

CHAPTER ONE **7**
Introducing Ebola

CHAPTER TWO **21**
Emergence

CHAPTER THREE **35**
Management of Deadly Disease

CHAPTER FOUR **46**
Level 4 Biohazard

CHAPTER FIVE **55**
The Impact of Ebola

GLOSSARY **66**

FOR MORE INFORMATION **70**

FOR FURTHER READING **74**

BIBLIOGRAPHY **75**

INDEX **77**

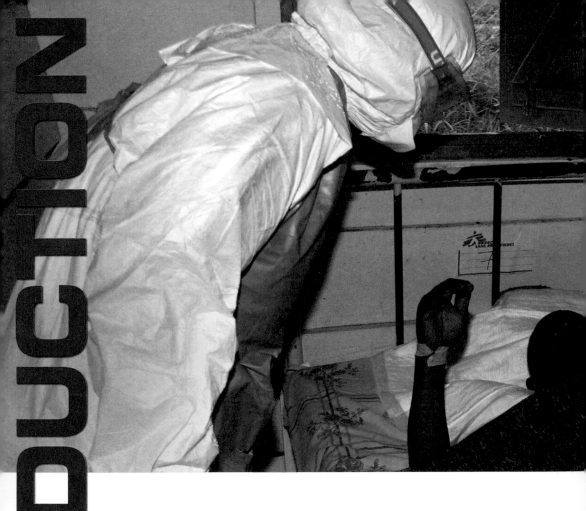

INTRODUCTION

"Epidemic" is a term that describes the spread of a disease in much higher numbers and with much wider reach than is expected. Usually, these localized occurrences involve illnesses that are not very serious or that resolve on their own, like the flu or a stomach bug. Sometimes, however, these illnesses keep spreading, either because scientists and doctors haven't figured out how they are transmitted or because they are unable to control the spread. In these cases, diseases can spread outside a localized area and run the risk of becoming a more global problem, or a pandemic, an illness that affects a whole region, continent, or even the world.

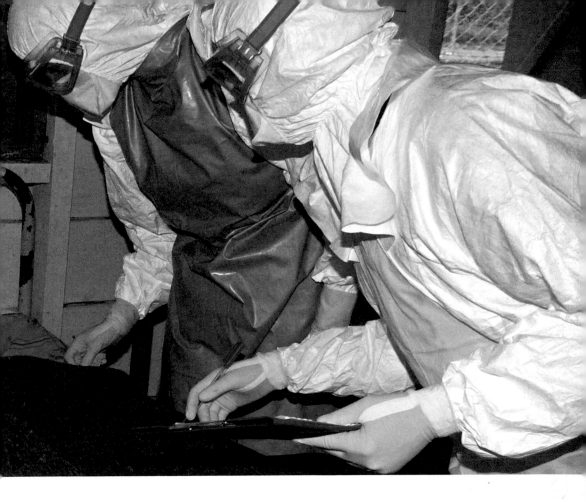

Members of a Swiss medical team, covered from head to toe in bio-protective gear, examine a terrified man suspected of carrying a new strain of Ebola during an outbreak in Bundibugyo, Uganda, in 2007.

In August 1976, in the town of Yambuku and a number of neighboring villages in Central Africa's Democratic Republic of the Congo (formerly Zaire), a very mysterious illness appeared. Its initial symptoms were unremarkable enough: a mild headache followed by a high fever with some nausea and vomiting. However, the disease rapidly progressed to confusion, weakness, and terrible pain as the lining of the body's blood vessels and internal organs began to break down and bleed uncontrollably. The victims' blood lost its ability to clot, resulting in streaming bloody gums and noses, bloody projectile vomit, and bloody diarrhea. Their internal organs stopped working. Their lungs filled with blood that was coughed out in spatters. Victims reportedly bled from their eyes and from the skin itself. The only mercy the virus showed was that the victims sometimes descended into a state of dementia, in which they had little awareness of their condition before their exhausted and ravaged bodies succumbed to the illness—all within roughly ten days from the onset of symptoms.

This terrible illness—which was named Ebola hemorrhagic fever after the Ebola River in Zaire—became more than a disease feared by locals. In fact, Ebola became a concern to scientists around the world who feared the illness might spread globally and kill hundreds of thousands of people. Because of its vague initial symptoms that are easily mistaken for other less serious illnesses, Ebola was often not recognized in time to contain it. Additionally, no one knew how it spread, where it came from, or how to cure it. As a result, Ebola caused tremendous panic. Although we now know that Ebola is caused by a virus, to this day many mysteries remain: where the virus comes from, how to cure it, and why some victims survive and others do not. Ebola, like HIV/AIDS and swine flu, is an emerging infectious disease. This means that while the Ebola virus may not be a new virus, the illness it causes has suddenly appeared in places it didn't exist before, thus posing a potentially serious risk to the health of human beings.

CHAPTER ONE

INTRODUCING EBOLA

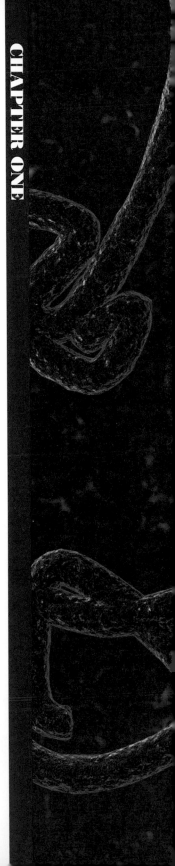

The Ebola virus cannot be seen with an ordinary microscope. In fact, the Ebola virus is so small that more than ten thousand viruses (or viral particles) could fit on the period at the end of this sentence. As a result, the virus can only be viewed with an electron microscope, which uses a concentrated beam of electrons. An electron microscope can magnify objects up to two million times their size, whereas a light microscope only achieves magnification of up to two thousand times.

Ebola is a virus of both human and non-human primates (such as chimpanzees, monkeys, and gorillas). Viruses are microscopic biological agents that infect the cells of other organisms where they replicate, or make more of themselves. Without these host cells, a virus can do nothing. In other words, viruses depend upon their hosts for survival. For example, if someone with the flu sneezed out one virus particle in an isolated room, that one virus would just sit there until it was somehow destroyed or until someone breathed it in. The influenza virus would then infect the healthy cells of the new host and use them to make more influenza viruses by taking over normal cellular function. When that host sneezes or coughs in the presence of another person who breathes in the virus, the process begins again.

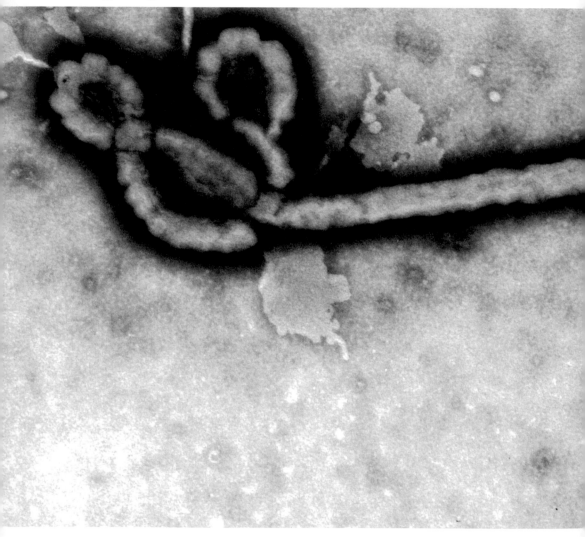

Imaging by the transmission electron microscope reveals the coiled, threadlike structure of the Ebola virus. Created by microbiologist Frederick A. Murphy in 1976, this image gave Ebola a face for the first time. Expecting to observe the Marburg virus, this image made it clear to scientists that they were dealing with an entirely new virus.

Biological Hijacking

All organisms contain coded genetic material that when "translated" is used to make all the proteins that an organism needs to survive. In other words, this material acts as a blueprint for building an organism. Human cells contain double-stranded coded material called DNA. Human cells decode DNA into single-stranded RNA, which is then used as a template to build human proteins. Viruses cannot make their own proteins. They need host cells to help them do it, and they must infect the cells of another organism in order to replicate. The Ebola virus is made up of genetic material that takes the form of another type of RNA, which it uses to trick the human cells it infects into making the proteins required to make more of the virus.

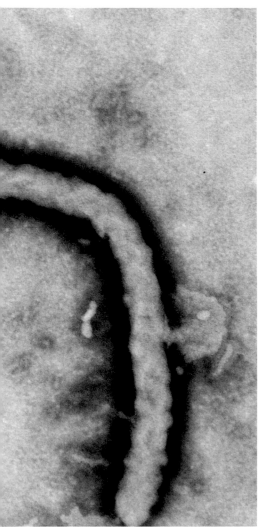

Ebola enters a human cell by using one of seven surface proteins to trick the cell into thinking the virus is not harmful, thereby evading detection by the human immune system that would otherwise destroy it. Once inside the cell, the virus turns its negative RNA into millions of copies of positive RNA, which the cell then treats as it would its own positive RNA; it is used to build proteins. Instead of building human proteins, however, the infected cell starts making virus proteins. These proteins are then put together to make more whole viruses. In other words, the virus turns infected cells into virus factories. In this way, one virus can become millions of viruses in a relatively short amount of time. This process of exponential replication is one key to a virus's survival. Eventually, an infected cell becomes packed with new viruses, which are released and go on to infect healthy neighboring cells, where the process starts again. This process continues until the body manages to mount an immune response to fight the virus, or, as is usually the case with Ebola, the person dies because

The "Thread" Viruses

There are several types of viruses, and they are divided into families. The Ebola virus belongs to the virus family Filoviridae, which means "thread virus." This is because the Ebola virus looks like a long string, usually with loops on one end. Scientists have called the shape a Cheerio with a tail, or, more commonly, a shepherd's crook. The Marburg virus, the other member of the Filoviridae family, looks similar under an electron microscope. Worldwide, seeing a virus of this shape under a microscope when it is not expected causes terrible panic in a lab.

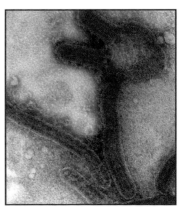

The Marburg virus, the only known relative of the Ebola virus, is viewed by transmission electron microscopy in 1968.

the damage that the virus causes overwhelms the body's ability to function.

Unknown Hiding Place

Every infectious agent, including protozoa, bacteria, and viruses, has a reservoir, a natural habitat in which it lives without causing harm, such as a jungle ecosystem or even inside a certain type of animal. A vector is the vehicle that transmits the disease from its natural reservoir to a new host where it can multiply. Vectors are often animals or insects that carry the infectious agent without getting sick themselves and transmit it to other hosts. For example, the reservoir for the bacteria that causes Lyme disease is a type of mouse, and its vector is an insect called a tick. The tick picks up the Lyme bacteria from biting a mouse, and then when the tick bites a human, it transmits the bacteria to its new host. In human hosts, which are not natural reservoirs, these bacteria cause an illness. In the case of illnesses like Lyme disease, scientists know exactly how the disease is spread and therefore know how it can be prevented.

The reservoir of the Ebola virus, however, is still unknown despite years of research. Scientists have tested hundreds of animal and insect species, including bats, spiders, bedbugs, rats, mice, squirrels, pigs, cows, mosquitoes, reptiles, and even antelope, but none has contained the virus. This is one of the most alarming factors about the Ebola virus. Because scientists have no idea where the Ebola virus originated or how each index case—the first known case of a new epidemic—became infected with it, they cannot tell people how to avoid it. It is thought to be zoonotic, or spread from animals to humans, based on the histories of the various index cases.

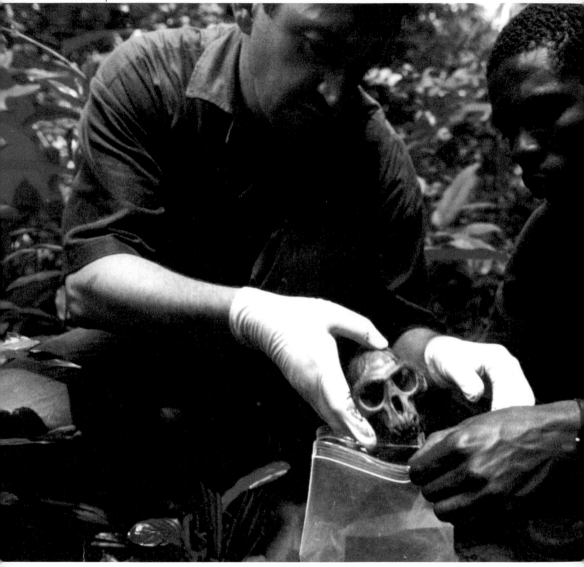

Researchers looking for the source of Ebola collect specimens in the jungles surrounding an area affected by the deadly virus. The reservoir, a carrier of the virus that does not suffer its ill effects but can spread the disease, is still unknown.

One theory is that the virus lives in certain African insects, such as spiders or mosquitoes that might be encountered on jungle hikes in remote areas. Other possibilities are that Ebola lives in African rodents or nonhuman primates to which hunters

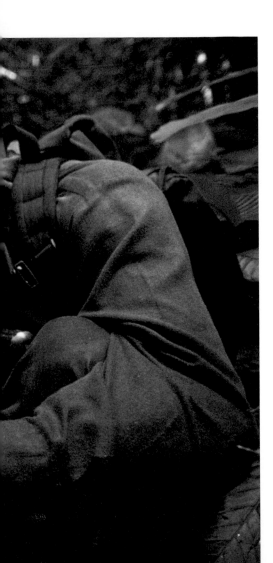

or monkey traders might be exposed. The Ebola-Zaire index case, a man named Mabalo, had purchased and eaten antelope meat fifty miles (eighty kilometers) from Yambuku, but no other cases have been traced to antelope. One current theory is that the Ebola virus may live inside certain African fruit bats that might take refuge in caves or old factories. This theory originates from the fact that when these bats were infected with Ebola in laboratory settings, they did not become ill, as most other lab animals did. This would make them excellent candidates for maintaining the virus in rainforests of the Bumba Zone. Thus far, however, no studies have revealed the true hiding place of Ebola. The only thing scientists know is that the index case in each new Ebola outbreak is exposed to something from which the virus is unknowingly picked up and brought home.

It is also important to note that just because a virus suddenly appears does not necessarily mean it is new. It is entirely possible that Ebola, as well as other emerging viruses, is older than humans. Ebola, for example, may have been hiding in the jungles of Africa for centuries. As human society continues to expand due to population growth and depletion of natural resources in overpopulated areas, people are forced to venture deeper into previously unexplored areas where they may stumble upon the reservoir of viruses like Ebola.

It is equally possible that Ebola has existed in the immediate vicinity of humans in Africa for some time, but that it recently mutated, or changed, in such a way that enabled it to infect humans. Many viruses mutate frequently, including the influenza virus. That is the reason why the flu vaccine must be updated with new viral strains each year; last year's flu vaccine will not provide protection from newer, mutated versions of the virus. Viral mutation is currently a topic of much interest. Swine flu, a form of influenza that normally infects pigs, is known to have only recently mutated to a form that can infect human beings.

Routes of Infection

The way that a virus gets from one host to another is known as its mode of transmission. For example, the influenza virus's mode of transmission is typically through inhalation of the airborne virus from an infected person's sneeze or cough. Ebola's mode of transmission is different, however. It is certain that exposure to infected blood, organs, and bodily secretions has been responsible for the person-to-person spread of the Ebola virus.

For example, a doctor working to save a patient who is violently coughing and vomiting blood may contract Ebola by accidentally ingesting the virus. As a result, family members caring for Ebola-stricken individuals are also at risk for being infected with the Ebola virus. We know that preparation of a body for funeral rites has resulted in transmission of Ebola from the infected body to the person preparing the body, perhaps through breaks in the preparer's skin. It is also thought that animal-to-person transmission can occur. This was likely the cause of infection in cases where a person dissected infected monkeys or handled or ate other infected mammals, including an African antelope. The risk of transmission of Ebola is made even higher by the fact that the Ebola virus replicates so rapidly that it effectively turns the victim's body into a "virus bomb." The victim's blood becomes so loaded with viruses—a condition called viremia—that exposure to even a milliliter of infected blood exposes a person to up to a million Ebola virus particles.

In addition, Ebola has mostly infected people who live in very poor, underprivileged villages, towns, and cities. Local hospitals often are ill equipped to handle large numbers of patients, forcing them into close quarters and increasing the risk of exposure to the virus. Usually, these hospitals cannot afford protective gowns, masks, or even running water in which to wash hands, bedding, and equipment. They are often unable to purchase new medical equipment and must reuse needles and syringes in order to serve their patients. Often, these items are not cleaned properly or at all between patients due to a lack of money to adequately sterilize medical equipment. Therefore, if a patient with Ebola is given an injection, the next patient on whom that needle is used is at very high risk of being infected with the Ebola virus and developing Ebola disease.

This kind of hospital-caused spread of disease is known as nosocomial infection. Nosocomial infection of hospital patients, particularly with disease-causing bacteria, is a huge problem worldwide. In many cases, however, these circumstances are a product of desperation, lack of resources, and extreme poverty

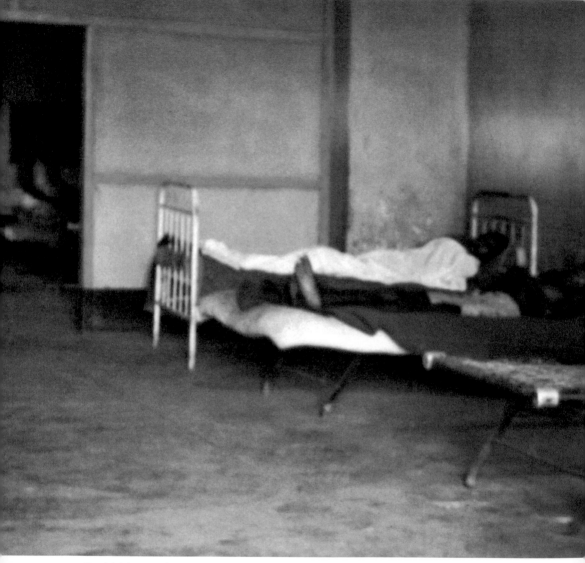

Bedridden patients lie in a Sudanese hospital during the 1976 Ebola outbreak. In these small, financially struggling rural hospitals, patients often share close quarters, greatly increasing the risk of spreading the virus to others, including hospital workers.

and not simply poor medical practice. These facilities must do the best they can with what little they have.

The viruses that cause the flu and common cold are spread via air, and there has been some concern that, under very

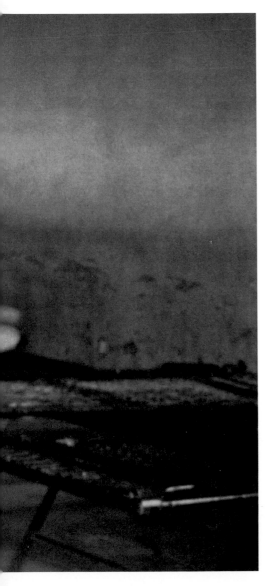

specific circumstances, Ebola may also be spread by this route. This is a terrifying thought because if the Ebola virus could be transmitted through the air, it would spread much faster and much farther, particularly given the fact that international travel, by car, by sea, and by air, has made airborne diseases much more difficult to contain. Thus far, it appears that no humans have been infected with Ebola by breathing it in nonlaboratory settings, such as hospitals or homes. However, like other viruses, Ebola may have the potential to mutate to a form that might one day be spread by air. In fact, there is some question whether this may have already occurred in laboratory settings among monkeys.

A Ticking Time Bomb

The time it takes from the moment a person is infected by an infectious agent, like a virus, to the moment symptoms are first experienced is known as the incubation period. If you were to come into contact with someone who has the flu, you would likely become ill within one to three days, the incubation period of influenza. However, the Ebola virus has a much wider range of incubation, from two to twenty-one days. During this time, the risk of spreading the illness is low. The onset of symptoms is usually sudden, but may begin with subtle symptoms that are vague, easily ignored, or attributable to something else. These initial symptoms are generally fever, joint and muscle aches, headache, sore throat, and weakness. These are all common complaints that are seen with numerous other illnesses, most of which are harmless, and patients are frequently sent home to rest or treated for malaria, a common illness in the areas in which Ebola has surfaced.

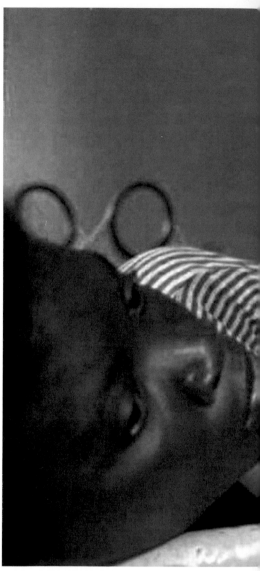

Unfortunately, once a person with Ebola has a fever, he or she is considered contagious, or able to spread the virus to others. If a patient is sent home during this period of nonspecific complaints, or if he or she is kept in the hospital around other patients, the risk of spreading the virus becomes increasingly higher as the patient becomes sicker. The highest risk of transmission occurs when the patient develops a rash, begins vomiting, having diarrhea, or "bleeds out." Bleeding out is a very late stage of Ebola that occurs

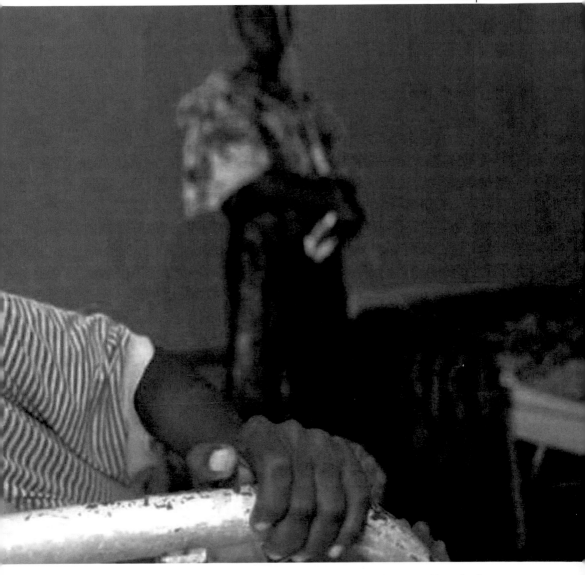

A young woman suffering from high fever, bloody diarrhea, and headache, classic symptoms of the Ebola virus, waits in the emergency room of Kikwit General Hospital.

because the linings of the patient's blood vessels and organs have broken down due to all the infected and ruptured cells. Like a hose punched with thousands of tiny holes, the vessels cannot contain the blood within them, and they seep and ooze.

Eventually, the patient's lungs and stomach fill with blood, leading to fits of bloody, virus-loaded coughs and vomiting. Blood leaks into the skin and gums, resulting in deep purple bruises. Sometimes, blood even leaks through the pores of the skin. Usually, the patient's nose bleeds uncontrollably and the whites of his or her eyes become deep red as vessels lose their integrity. Sadly, because this bleeding occurs in the fragile brain tissue as well, many patients with late-stage Ebola become dazed (stuporous), silently stare off into space and are unable to recognize family or friends, develop hallucinations, or become hysterical and appear crazy. Because of all the bleeding it causes, Ebola has been described as a hemorrhagic fever.

CHAPTER TWO

EMERGENCE

The Congo rainforest in the present Democratic Republic of the Congo in Central Africa is the second largest rainforest in the world, accounting for 18 percent of the planet's remaining rainforest. More than six hundred tree species and ten thousand animal species inhabit the area. In fact, much of the Congo rainforest remains unexplored. Through this forest flows the mighty Congo River.

The river and jungle make up one of the world's most important and fragile ecosystems, a group of living organisms that, coupled with their physical environment, function as a unit. In recent decades, increasing deforestation has greatly disrupted the natural balance in the Congo. It has disturbed the homes of animals and plant species, and it has forced humans and animals to venture deeper into the uncharted forest in search of food and, in the case of humans, items to trade. In so doing, humans and animals may come into contact with several yet undiscovered species of animals, plants, and microorganisms, some of which may cause illness or even death. On returning home from hunting, foraging, or exploring, humans may bring these microorganisms with them, exposing anyone they have contact with to infection.

The First Case

In 1976, after two weeks of travel in the Mobayi-Mbongo Zone, an equatorial town in a northern jungle region of Africa, forty-four-year-old Mabalo Lokela visited the Yambuku Mission Hospital with a headache that he was sure was due to another case of malaria. Though it served more than sixty thousand patients, the hospital was small, staffed by nuns with no formal medical training, and medical equipment was in short supply due to poverty. Only five needles and syringes were issued each morning to staff, and these were rinsed between patients in a pan of warm water.

Mabalo received a quinine injection, a dated but common treatment for malaria—a blood disease spread by mosquitoes—and was sent home to his wife. At the same time, a young female was receiving blood transfusions for anemia—a deficiency of red blood cells—and another was recovering from malaria, tended to by her husband. In another ward, an older man was recovering from surgery. His wife, at his bedside, received multiple vitamin injections to aid her exhaustion.

Two days later, a thirty-year-old man arrived complaining of diarrhea and a severe bloody nose. His symptoms were mysterious, and despite various injections the patient did not improve. Bleeding heavily from his nose, he left the hospital against the wishes of the nuns who were baffled by his illness. All of these patients, including Mabalo, had received injections with needles that were reused, that had not been properly sterilized, and that therefore harbored a deadly pathogen.

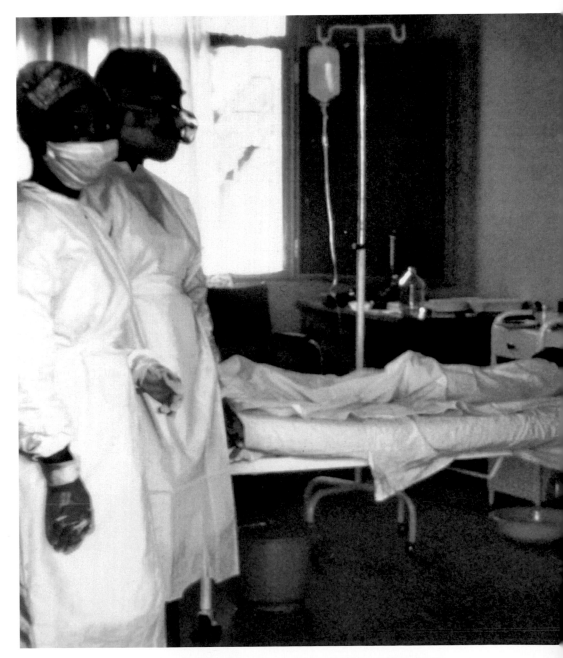

Health care workers wearing protective gear at Ngaliema Hospital in Kinshasa, Zaire, watch over an Ebola patient in the final stages of the illness. This patient later succumbed to the virus despite aggressive attempts to save her.

Of course, none of this was known by the overworked nuns who did their best to treat their patients.

Types of Ebola

Just as there are different breeds of dog, such as the poodle and German shepherd, the Ebola virus has different strains. There are currently five known Ebola strains, each with slightly different characteristics and each named for the geographic area in which it emerged.

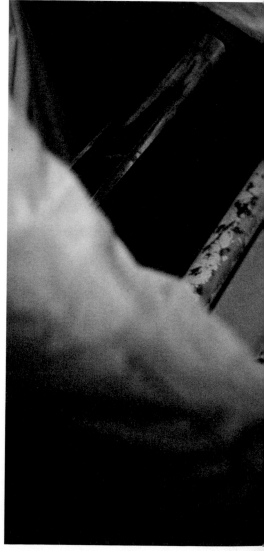

The first to be recognized was Ebola-Zaire, for which Mabalo Lokela was the index case. The second was Ebola-Sudan, for which the cotton factory worker in Nzara was the index case. The third, Ebola-Reston, is the only Ebola virus to be found outside of Africa. It was named for Reston, Virginia, the site of a quarantine facility where crab-eating monkeys imported from the Philippines fell ill with the virus. To this day, no humans have fallen ill due to Ebola-Reston. The fourth, Ebola–Ivory Coast, sickened one scientist who performed an autopsy on a wild chimpanzee in the forest. The fifth and most recently discovered strain of Ebola is Ebola-Bundibugyo, named after the site of a 2007 Ebola outbreak in Uganda, which borders both Sudan and Zaire (now the Democratic Republic of the Congo). During this outbreak, 149 people fell ill and 25 percent died. This makes

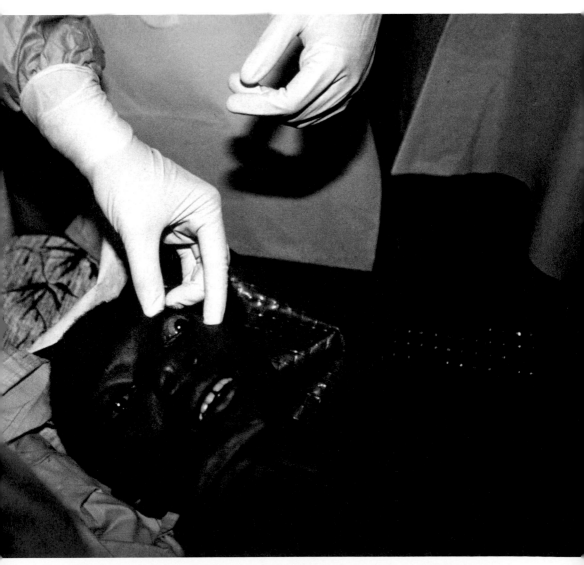

The whites of the eyes often become bright red in patients suffering from Ebola, as small blood vessels become porous, causing blood to leak out into the surrounding tissues. For this reason, Ebola is known as a hemorrhagic illness.

Ebola-Zaire, the strain responsible for Ebola's initial recognition, the deadliest of the Ebola strains.

No one knows how many Ebola strains truly exist. There may be several more or just these five. But if the virus mutates, as many viruses do, different strains can still emerge. These may be more or less dangerous than those we currently know of. Thus far, all of the known outbreaks with all strains have occurred abruptly, with no known sources, and with subsequent spread between people or between species of nonhuman primate.

Six days after his initial quinine injection, Mabalo Lokela returned to the hospital with a high fever. Though his condition was unusual, he was sent home to be cared for by his wife. He returned within days, critically ill. He had developed bloody diarrhea and was vomiting blood. His eyes appeared sunken due to severe dehydration. He was confused, agitated, and suffered from high fever and headache. His nose bled. His gums bled. Unbeknownst to the Mission Hospital staff, the anemic woman who had returned home after her blood transfusions suffered the same symptoms as Mabalo. Her sister who had cared for her also developed fever and headache. Also back home, the young woman recovering from malaria was very ill. Her husband was vomiting and bleeding from his eyes. And the young wife who had received vitamin injections during her husband's surgical recovery was now delirious and hemorrhaging blood. Eventually, all of them died.

On September 8, ten days after he first came to the hospital, Mabalo Lokela died a terrible, painful death despite treatment with antibiotics, vitamins, chloroquine, and fluids. He is now known as Ebola's index case for Ebola-Zaire. His body was prepared for burial in the customary way, which involved the removal of food and excreta from his body by the bare hands of the women in his family.

Ebola Timeline and Map of Incidence

Year	Ebola strain	Location	Human cases	Death rate	History
1976	Ebola-Zaire	Yambuku, DRC	318	88 percent	First time Ebola is seen. Infection spread by close contact with victims and shared needles in hospital setting.
1976	Ebola-Sudan	Nzara, Sudan	284	53 percent	First victim a cotton factory worker. No link to Ebola cases in Zaire.
1976	Ebola-Sudan	England	1	0 percent	Lab infection; accidental con-tamination via needle stick.
1979	Ebola-Sudan	Nzara, Sudan	34	65 percent	Same site as previous outbreak in Sudan.
1989–1992	Ebola-Reston	USA/Italy	0	0 percent	Ebola introduced to quarantined labs by monkeys imported from the Philippines. No human cases, but represents the ease with which the virus could spread globally.
1994	Ebola-Zaire	Gabon	44	63 percent	In rainforest, assumed to be yellow fever. Identified as Ebola in 1995.
1994	Ebola-Ivory Coast	Ivory Coast	1	0 percent	Researcher ill after autopsy on wild chimpanzee.

Year	Ebola strain	Location	Human cases	Death rate	History
1995	Ebola-Zaire	DRC	315	81 percent	First case in patient who worked in nearby forest.
1996	Ebola-Zaire	Gabon	37	57 percent	Chimp found dead in forest and eaten by hunters. Cases were those involved in butchering and their families.
1996	Ebola-Zaire	Gabon	60	75 percent	First case in hunter living in forest, spread by close contact. Dead chimp found in area where first case was infected.
1996	Ebola-Zaire	South Africa	2	50 percent	Medical worker who treated infected patients in Gabon brings Ebola to Johannesburg. The nurse who cared for him died.
1996	Ebola-Reston	USA	0	0 percent	Infected monkey from Philippines. No human cases.
2000–2001	Ebola-Sudan	Uganda	425	53 percent	Largest outbreak. Risk highest in those attending funerals of Ebola victims, having family contact with Ebola victims, and providing medical care to Ebola patients without adequate protective gear.
2001–2002	Ebola-Zaire	Gabon/DRC	122	79 percent	Outbreak along border of two nations.

Year	Ebola strain	Location	Human cases	Death rate	History
2002–2003	Ebola-Zaire	DRC	143	89 percent	Outbreaks in the districts of Mbomo and Kéllé.
2003	Ebola-Zaire	DRC	35	29 percent	Outbreak in villages of Mbomo and Mbandza in Mbomo district.
2004	Ebola-Sudan	Sudan	17	41 percent	Outbreak in Yambio county in southern Sudan at same time as a measles out-break. Many cases originally suspected to be Ebola were later classified as measles.
2007	Ebola-Zaire	DRC	249	78 percent	Outbreak in Kasai Occidental Province.
2007	Ebola-Bundibugyo	Uganda	139	25 percent	First reported occurrence of new, fifth strain.

Abbreviations: DRC — Democratic Republic of the Congo (formerly Zaire)

Contagion

Many people attended Mabalo Lokela's funeral. Within a week, his wife (who was pregnant), sister, mother, mother-in-law, and his wife's sister all developed the same symptoms. Only his wife and her sister survived. The rest, including his unborn child, succumbed to the illness.

The disease began to spread more rapidly though Yambuku, killing more than two-thirds of its victims. No medications worked, the hospitals ran out of supplies, and needles continued to be reused. Hospitals had no choice, given the short supply of needles and the relative poverty of the area. People began to panic. Desperate, the others radioed a doctor in a town 50 miles (80 km) away. The doctor came to Yambuku immediately.

Eventually, one of the four nuns at the hospital fell ill. Horrified by what he saw at the mission hospital, Dr. Ngoi

Marburg

When researcher Peter Piot viewed the image through his electron microscope, his heart skipped a beat. What he saw reminded him all too much of another deadly hemorrhagic virus known as Marburg. Marburg was identified in 1967, when a group of researchers working with Ugandan monkeys fell ill after handling tissues from the primates. Seven of the thirty-one individuals who were infected with the virus died. Shortly thereafter, Marburg was recognized in isolated outbreaks throughout Africa, none of which led to a massive eruption like the Ebola epidemics seen in Yambuku and Nzara.

Still, scientists thought it was possible that Marburg might be responsible for the new outbreaks and that antiserum collected from past Marburg victims might help new victims fight the illness. Antiserum is made from the blood of a person who has been infected with a disease and survived. It contains antibodies that can fight against a disease, and the researchers hoped it could prevent a newly infected person from becoming ill.

Though the idea was a good one, the Marburg antiserum did not save the patients falling ill in Zaire and Sudan. They continued to die and the disease continued to spread. This was the first evidence that the disease erupting through these regions was not Marburg, but a never-before-seen, even more deadly hemorrhagic disease. This both excited and terrified researchers around the world. Eventually, this virus came to be known as Ebola, after the Ebola River in Zaire.

Mushola called for the use of antiseptic measures, including boiling water and sterilizing medical instruments. He also recommended that the locals change their funeral and burial practices despite long-standing customs. He also contacted the capital city of Kinshasa, which sent an epidemiologist—someone who studies how to control the spread of disease—and a microbiologist—someone who studies the agents that cause disease—directly to Yambuku.

Alarmed by the horrible death of an infected infant right before their eyes, the researchers cut their planned six-day trip to twenty-four hours. In that time, they took samples of the victims' blood, tissues, and organs to study in Kinshasa. They also brought Myriam, a nurse who had developed symptoms, back with them in the hopes that resources at the larger Kinshasa hospital would help her. Unfortunately, they could not save her. Myriam died on September 30, and the disease spread to Mayinga, the nurse who cared for her. Still, no one knew what the disease was or how to stop it.

Containment, Quarantine, and New Outbreaks

Given the rapid spread and deadly nature of the mysterious new disease that would come to be known as Ebola, Dr. Ngwete Kikhela, the Kinshasan Minister of Health, and Zaire President Mobutu Sese Seko declared the entire Bumba Zone, which includes Yambuku and Kinshasa, a quarantine zone to prevent further spread of the illness. No one was permitted to enter or leave the area. Roads, waterways, and airfields came under martial law. Children were kept home from school, community and social events were postponed, and businesses closed.

While the disease spread in Zaire, reports surfaced of similar illnesses in two rural, impoverished towns in southern

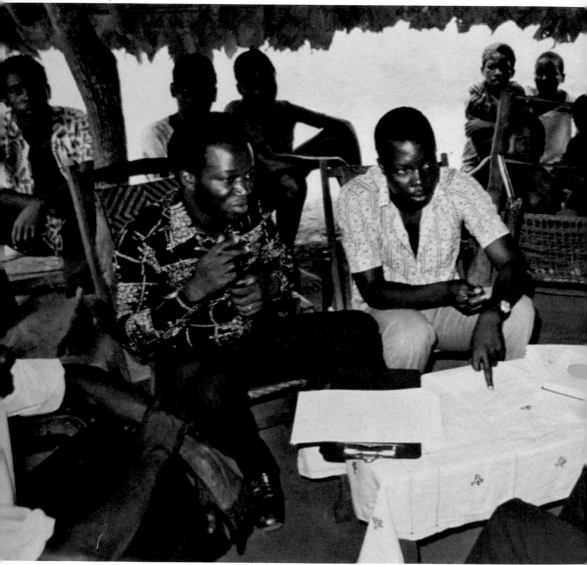

Health officials in what is now the Democratic Republic of the Congo gather to discuss data collected during the nation's 1976 Ebola outbreak in the hopes of controlling the spread of the virus.

Sudan, roughly 500 miles (800 km) from Yambuku. This illness was traced back to a man—now recognized as the index case for Ebola-Sudan—who worked in a factory in Nzara that made cloth out of raw cotton. This man and two coworkers who

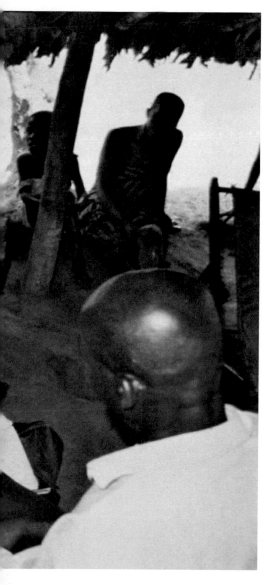

also fell ill somehow transmitted the illness to a club owner who, when he developed symptoms, had the money to travel to a hospital in the city of Maridi. As in the Yambuku Mission Hospital, it was there that the Ebola virus spread rapidly. Interestingly, no definitive link was ever found between the two outbreaks.

When all was said and done, the Ebola outbreak in Zaire claimed 280 lives out of 318 cases, a striking 88 percent of its victims. The Sudan outbreak was only slightly less deadly, claiming the lives of 151 of its 284 victims, or 53 percent. By comparison, of the millions of individuals in the United States who become infected with the influenza virus each year, the illness claims only an estimated thirty-six thousand people. After the initial outbreak, there were few outbreaks over the next few years, and then the Ebola virus disappeared as mysteriously as it came and was not seen again for more than a decade.

Since 1989, Ebola has made other short-lived appearances, including another large outbreak in Uganda, which borders both Sudan and the area formerly called Zaire. All

Ugandan hospital workers are on their way to bury an Ebola victim. Disposal of Ebola-infected bodies poses an issue in many nations, as customary funeral rites often involve exposure to infected bodily fluids and organs, resulting in transmission of the virus to others.

outbreaks were limited to relatively small geographic areas in Africa, and none were as deadly as the one that began at the Yambuku Mission Hospital in 1976. Nonetheless, the possibility of another epidemic, or worse, a pandemic if an Ebola outbreak is not contained, strikes fear in the hearts of scientists because no one is any closer to understanding Ebola's origin or how to cure it.

MANAGEMENT OF DEADLY DISEASE

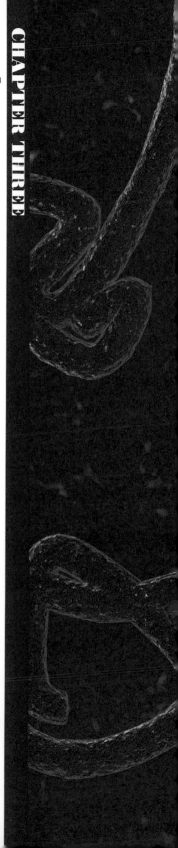

Human males and females of any age are susceptible to the Ebola virus, though it is unclear why some people survive the ravages of the disease and others do not. It is also known that many species of nonhuman primates are also susceptible, including the crab-eating monkeys that came to the Reston lab and died in droves, and the wild chimpanzee that a scientist dissected while exploring the Ivory Coast. Research has indicated that in 2007, thousands of gorillas and chimpanzees died from Ebola having eaten from the same fruit trees, though at different times. It is thought that they came in contact with infected bodily fluids at the fruit trees.

In fact, Ebola has reportedly killed one-quarter of the earth's gorilla population. These facts also make it unlikely that nonhuman primates are the long sought after reservoir. These animals, like humans, are also host organisms, where the virus replicates and has its deadly effects. In experiments to find out more about Ebola, scientists have discovered that rabbits do not become ill if injected with Ebola, and guinea pigs only become slightly ill.

Diagnosing Ebola

Most people infected with Ebola carry very high concentrations of the virus in their blood. Specialized blood tests exist that can accurately detect if someone has been infected with the virus. These tests can be performed once the patient develops symptoms, after recovery, or even after death.

These tests are extremely important when new outbreaks occur, as researchers want to know without a doubt what is causing an illness so that they can better control its spread. However, for a number of reasons, most of these tests are not routinely performed in the areas in which Ebola outbreaks occur.

First, these are all small, rural, underprivileged areas that cannot afford the kinds of equipment and facilities that are necessary to conduct such tests. They are also not able to communicate readily with larger institutions that can test patients. In these areas, once an Ebola outbreak occurs, diagnoses are made clinically by looking at the patient's symptoms and listening to his or her story. Second, these patients usually die or are buried quickly before their blood or bodies can be sent to a facility that is able to test them for the virus or before researchers can arrive at the hospital to test patients themselves. The third and biggest reason why Ebola cannot be routinely tested for in just any hospital or lab is that the Ebola virus or Ebola-infected blood, tissues, or organs are simply too dangerous to be purposefully handled in routine laboratory settings.

In the United States, however, if someone were to develop symptoms of Ebola, testing would certainly be done. This is especially true if the patient had traveled to areas in which there have been outbreaks, or if they worked in labs that could put them at risk for contracting Ebola either from animals or blood samples. The United States and other developed nations

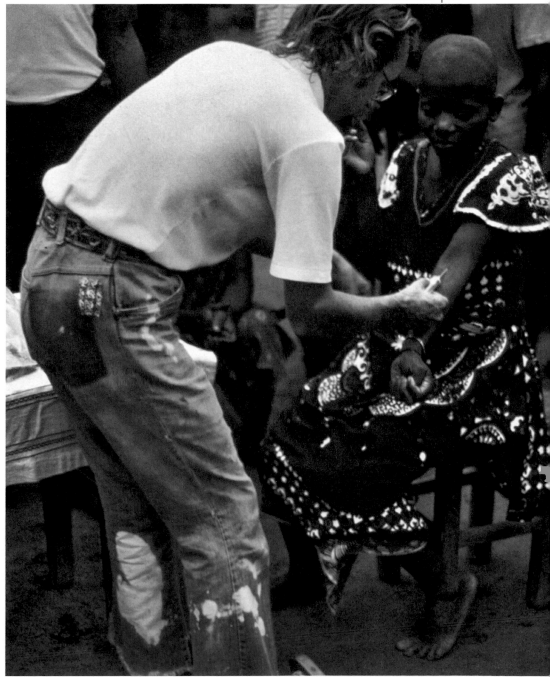

A member of an Ebola surveillance team in Yambuku, Zaire, takes blood samples from a village resident during the 1976 Ebola outbreak. Several villagers were tested for active Ebola infection but also for antibodies to the virus, indicating previous infection, but recovery.

are fortunate enough to have the financial and technical resources to perform this kind of testing in a timely and, most importantly, safe manner.

New Research

Vaccines are arguably the sin-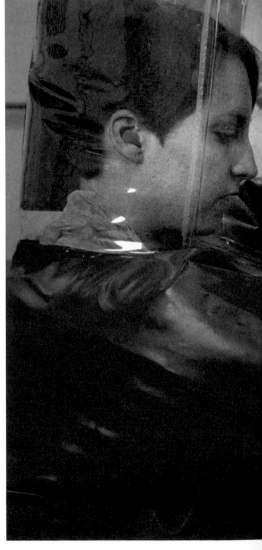
gle most important biomedical
achievement in the past cen-
tury. Before vaccines became
available and widely used,
humans were susceptible to a
wide range of deadly and debil-
itating illnesses, including polio
and measles. If you have not
heard of these illnesses, it is
most likely because they are
now considered, in developed
nations, to be of little concern.
This is because vaccines were
developed that immunize, or
protect, people against these
infections.

These diseases have not
disappeared from the planet,
however. Several countries
without adequate financial and
medical resources still struggle
with some of these vaccine-
preventable illnesses. In
addition, there have been increasing numbers of people in developed nations where the vaccines are readily available— and often required by law—that have chosen not to be

vaccinated themselves or have opted against vaccinating their children. As a result, there has been a resurgence of some diseases, such as whooping cough, that haven't been routinely seen in developed nations in many years.

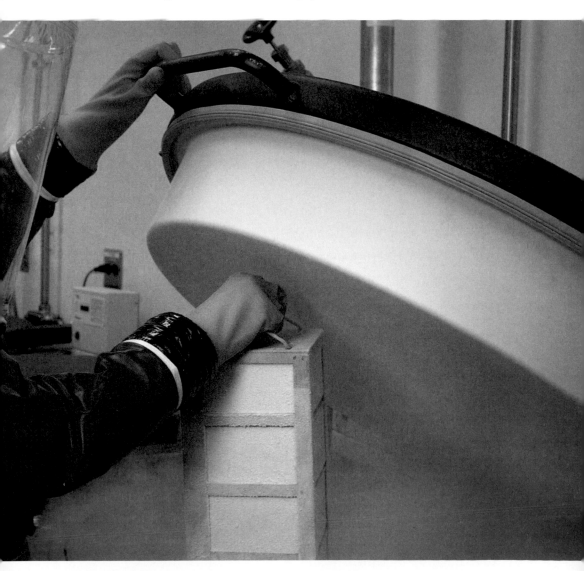

Wearing a Biosafety Level 4 positive pressure suit, a microbiologist with the Centers for Disease Control and Prevention's Special Pathogens Branch inserts a rack of highly infectious viral specimens into a liquid nitrogen freezer, where they can be safely stored for future research.

Vaccines contain either parts of viruses, "killed" whole viruses, or viruses that have been weakened to the point that they cannot infect a human being. All vaccines are designed to provoke an immune response by the body, including the production of specific antibodies to the infectious agent, without the person receiving the vaccine becoming ill.

Antibodies are the human immune system's specialized weapons against diseases. Once a person has sufficient antibodies to a virus, the virus can enter his or her body, but the person will not become ill because the antibodies to that virus will immediately recognize and kill it. Of course, if the virus mutates, the antibodies may no longer recognize the virus, and another vaccine must be developed to protect against this new form of the virus. This is the case with the influenza virus, which mutates rapidly, resulting in the need for new flu vaccines every year. However, viruses like polio mutate very slowly. As a result, polio vaccines are generally given only once in a person's life.

An Ebola Vaccine

Much research has gone into the development of an Ebola vaccine, and several experimental vaccines have been tested in recent years. This has been difficult given the kinds of labs required to handle Ebola and the small number of people that are specially trained to work in such environments. Unfortunately, "killed" virus vaccines, the safest type in the minds of researchers who are understandably reluctant to inject live or weakened versions of Ebola into the bloodstream of experimental subjects, have not shown promise.

In 2008, an Ebola vaccine shown to be effective in nonhuman primates was slated to be tested on people.

Treating Ebola

Despite the fact that scientists have aggressively been searching for a definitive treatment for Ebola, as well as a vaccine to prevent the virus from causing a deadly infection, the only treatments currently available to Ebola patients are known as supportive treatments. These generally involve treating the symptoms of an illness, rather than the illness itself until the patient either improves or dies.

In the case of Ebola, patients are kept hydrated with fluids, treated for any additional infections that occur while they are suffering, their oxygen levels and blood pressure are maintained, and medications are given to reduce pain. Treatment for symptoms caused by the influenza virus, which also has no cure, is also supportive. Treating the flu involves taking medications for headache and fever, drinking fluids, eating bland foods, and taking throat lozenges until the virus runs its course. Fortunately, unlike Ebola, most people with the flu do recover and supportive treatments merely help them stay comfortable along the way.

In March 2009, an experimental vaccine was used on a lab worker who accidentally stuck herself with a needle that was contaminated with Ebola. She never came down with the illness. It is unclear, however, whether the vaccine prevented the woman from developing the illness, or if the virus never entered her bloodstream. This means that there is no way to tell if the lab worker was simply lucky, or if the vaccine worked. This vaccine was made from another type of virus, but was designed to look like Ebola in the hopes that the antibodies produced from it would protect against the deadly virus. Such experimental vaccines are first tested in rodents, and then in nonhuman primates before they are tested in humans.

Experimental treatments for patients already infected with Ebola have involved substances that interfere with the virus's ability to multiply once it has entered the cells. Other treatments have been tested in rodents. In one experiment,

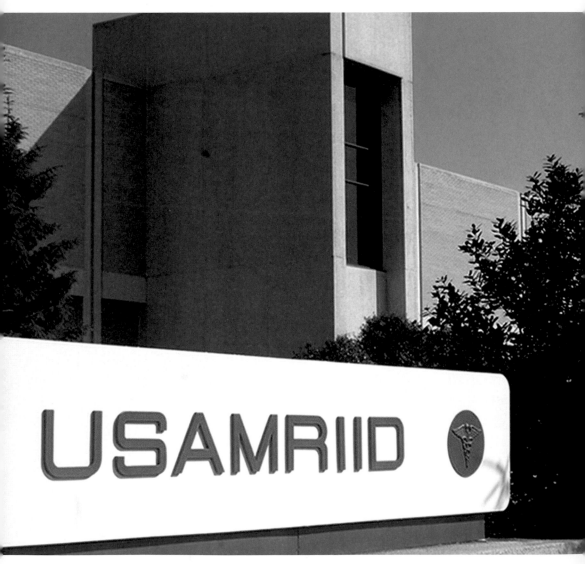

The lead medical research laboratory for the U.S. Biological Defense Research Program is the only laboratory in the Department of Defense equipped to safely study highly hazardous infectious agents requiring containment at Biosafety Level 4.

antibodies were extracted from mice that survived infection with Ebola and injected into other mice. When these mice were later exposed to Ebola, most of them survived. As has been done with Marburg, several experiments are being performed using antiserum from Ebola patients who miraculously survived infection in the hopes that their antibodies might be used to protect future victims.

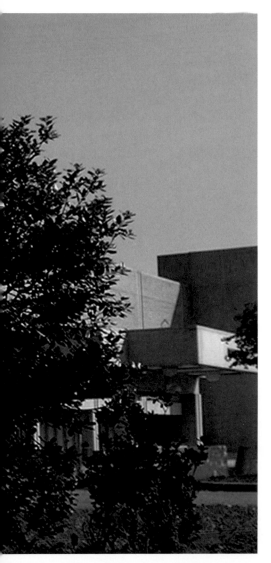

None of these experimental treatments or vaccines have been researched extensively enough to be used routinely. If any of them do show promise both in combating Ebola infection and being safe to use in humans, they will certainly be stockpiled in the event of an outbreak and delivered to areas of the globe in which Ebola is endemic or has been found naturally.

There has also been some interest in a tree that grows on the banks of the Ebola River known as *Garcinia kola*, which has long been used by traditional healers as a remedy for numerous ailments. In tests performed by the U.S. Army Medical Research Institute of Infectious Diseases (USAMRIID), extracts of this tree were shown to slow down the replication of Ebola in monkey cells placed in test tubes

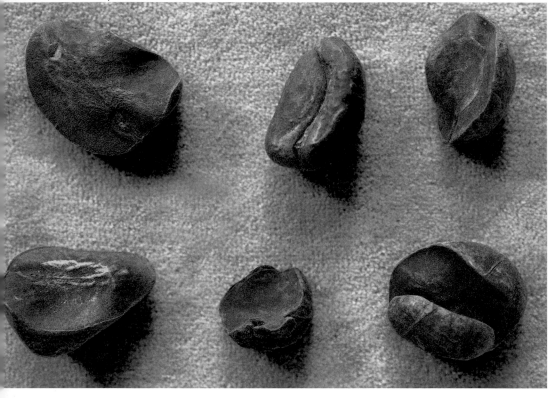

Garcinia kola has been shown in some animal studies to slow the replication of the Ebola virus. Scientists hope the plant may prove useful in the development of a cure or treatment for the deadly virus.

and petri dishes. The National Institutes of Health has funded the identification of forty-six potentially medicinal compounds from the *Garcinia kola* tree, and several experiments using these compounds have been performed. But thus far, few experiments on the plant's effect on the Ebola virus have been carried out.

Myths and Facts

MYTH The Ebola virus was engineered by scientists working to create the ultimate bioterrorism agent.

FACT While several conspiracy theories exist regarding the origins of Ebola, there is little evidence to support such a claim.

MYTH There have been human cases of Ebola in the United States.

FACT There have been no human cases of Ebola in the United States. The only cases were in imported laboratory monkeys, all of which were kept in quarantine. None of the lab workers became ill.

MYTH Ebola has become an airborne virus.

FACT There is no evidence yet that Ebola has become an airborne virus spread by respiratory droplets as is influenza or the common cold. Currently, Ebola is spread only by close contact with or ingestion of infected tissues, blood, and other bodily fluids.

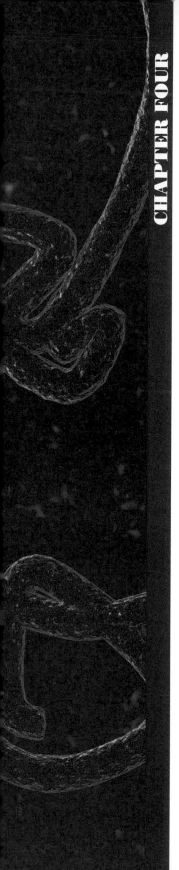

CHAPTER FOUR

LEVEL 4 BIOHAZARD

Ebola is often referred to in scientific slang as a "hot agent," given how deadly it is. For this reason, it is considered a Biosafety Level 4 virus. Biosafety Level 1 agents are those that are not known to cause illness in normally healthy humans. The lab in your school science classroom is a Level 1 lab. Biosafety Level 2 labs house agents that pose a moderate risk to people and the environment. Either vaccination to prevent illness by these Level 2 agents or antibiotics to treat illness caused by them are available in the event of exposure. An example of a Level 2 agent is measles, for which a vaccine is available. Biosafety Level 3 agents are those that cause serious or potentially lethal diseases if they are inhaled. These labs have high security, have two sets of doors, and are under negative pressure so that when doors to the outside open, air rushes in, not out, thereby containing the pathogens. The bacterium that causes tuberculosis, *Mycobacterium tuberculosis*, is an example of a Level 3 agent.

Level 4 agents like Ebola, however, are in a class all their own. Level 4 agents pose a very high risk of airborne infections and

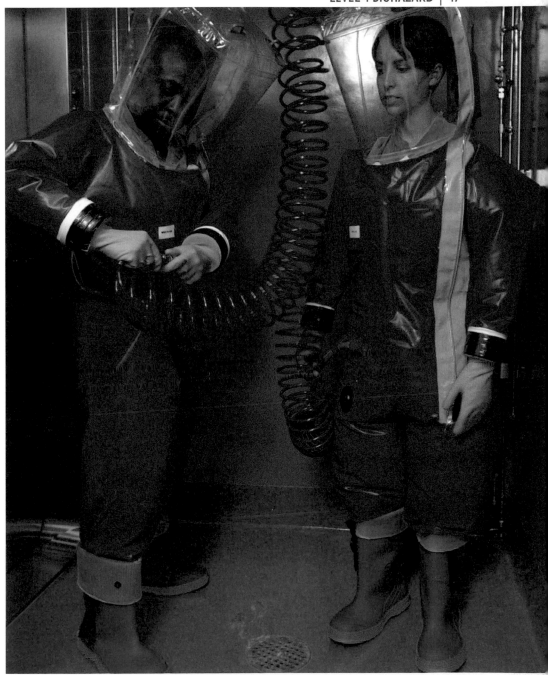

Microbiologists at the CDC suit up in preparation to enter a Biosafety
Level 4 laboratory, the only environment in which the Ebola virus can be
safely studied without risk of transmission to researchers.

life-threatening illness. These labs are in separate buildings or in highly controlled areas of other labs. Very few scientists are given clearance to work in these settings. No one with any immune system problems is permitted to work at Level 4 labs, and all workers must go through extensive blood tests and have their healthy serum collected and stored.

Like Level 3, these labs use negative pressure to prevent the outflow of contaminated air. Workers must take decontamination showers before they leave the lab and must walk through numerous air locks. No personal belongings are allowed in these labs. Everything researchers wear in a Level 4 area is provided by the lab, including socks and undergarments. They must also wear specially designed one-piece suits ventilated by a life support system with special air filters, alarms, and backup breathing tanks. The pressure inside the suit is higher than the pressure in the lab, so if a puncture occurs, clean air inside the suit will flow out into the contaminated environment instead of the other way around. Sharp instruments are restricted to use only when needed, and plastic serves as a substitute for glass. Numerous other safety precautions are also taken within these labs.

Biocontainment in the Environment

In real-world settings, particularly in small, underserved villages, like those in which Ebola outbreaks have occurred, such high-tech precautions are clearly impossible. But there are precautions that the people in such environments have learned to take to contain disease outbreaks, thereby controlling their spread to neighboring towns and villages.

When researchers, including Peter Piot and a member of the Centers for Disease Control and Prevention (CDC), came to Yambuku to assess the mysterious 1976 outbreak, what they

Viruses: Alive or Not?

One of the most long-standing debates in the history of biology is whether or not a virus is a living organism. Many scientists argue that they are not. Others contend that they are, and commonly accepted definitions of alive are too narrow and limited. According to many biologists, to be alive, organisms must fulfill basic life requirements. By this definition, living things are highly organized, complex structures; maintain a chemical composition that is different from their environment; have the capacity to take in, transform, and use energy from the environment (eating, drinking, metabolizing, and excreting waste); respond to stimuli; have the capacity to reproduce themselves; grow and evolve; and are well-suited to their environment.

As we have already learned, viruses are dependent on the cells of other organisms to reproduce; they cannot do so on their own. In addition, viruses do not eat, drink, excrete waste, or grow as other organisms do. Nor are they active in their environments with regard to responding to stimuli. This is the primary reason why viruses are considered by many to exist just at the border of living and nonliving. Some consider them nonliving parasites.

However, can scientists really draw a clear distinction between what is living and what is not? The current debate argues that the definition of life is not so simple as to be reduced to a list of criteria. For example, a rock is clearly not alive. Neither are the individual molecules that make up DNA, which is a template for the proteins that are required for life. But where does nonliving suddenly cross the line into living? While DNA and RNA viruses do not fulfill the basic life requirements, it is clear that they seek out certain cell types in their hosts and actively direct the host cell's machinery to produce new viruses.

encountered impressed them given the very limited resources the hardworking locals had at their fingertips. Already, the roads and waterways to and from the entire Bumba Zone had been shut down by the quarantine order of President Mobutu

Sese Seko, leaving them deserted and cutting the people of the area, as well as the virus, off from the rest of the world. The villages themselves, usually bustling with vendors, children, and various activities, were as quiet as ghost towns.

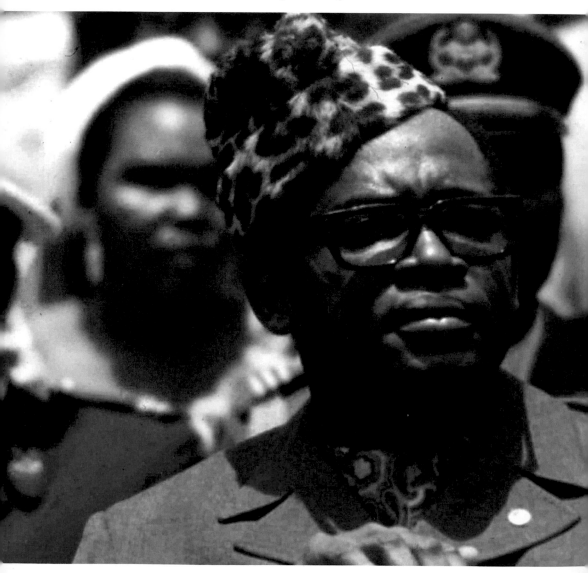

Zairian president Mobutu Sese Seko declared the area surrounding Yambuku and Kinshasa a quarantine zone during the first Ebola outbreak in 1976. No one was permitted to enter or leave the area in the hopes that the virus would burn itself out.

When the researchers approached the mission hospital, they found the building wrapped in strips of gauze, with hand-written signs warning people to stay away. A bell was hung at the entrance asking people to ring for assistance or leave their

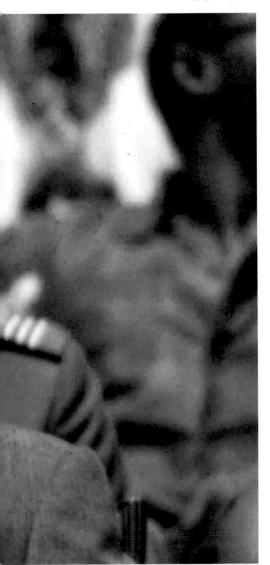

donations and depart quickly. When the researchers approached the entrance and rang the bell, the mission nuns came running, shouting, "Don't come near! You are going to die!"

The locals had erected roadblocks at the entrances of each village, all staffed by patrolmen around the clock. Traffic along the two local rivers, which served as a major source of imported goods, had come to a trickle. Villagers, ill and well, confined themselves to their homes. Few people traveled between neighboring villages. Patients suspected to be infected were isolated to specific areas. Dead bodies were buried at distances much farther than usual from living quarters and in communal cemeteries. The bodies were also wrapped in shrouds soaked in chemicals in attempts to kill whatever organisms were present. Chemicals, boiling, and burning were used to decontaminate or destroy contaminated clothing, utensils, and waste. Researchers who came to study the outbreak used respirators and goggles. More important, the administration of vaccinations and injections of any kind had been halted.

If there is no cure, what stopped the Ebola outbreaks in Zaire, Sudan, and those that followed? All of them slowed relatively quickly. The outbreak in Yambuku and the surrounding area lasted only twenty-six days. While exact reasons are not entirely understood, the precautions taken by the locals certainly helped contain the virus, as did the use of quarantines that prevented movement into and out of affected areas. Most important, the realization that reusing needles was the primary way the disease was spread and stopping this practice greatly stemmed the spread of Ebola.

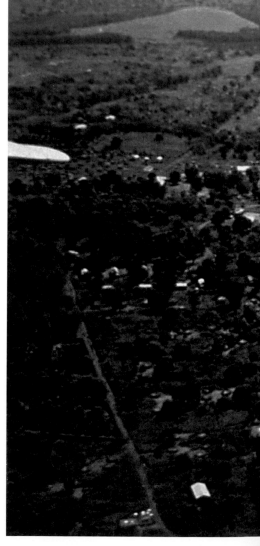

However, it may not simply be the actions of people that prevented Ebola from spreading so quickly across the African continent. Properties of the virus itself may have limited its potential to spread far and wide. As mentioned previously, the one purpose of a virus is to make more of itself. It does so by infecting various hosts, taking over their cells, and turning them into virus factories. A host must be alive to do this. If a virus is too deadly, it does itself a disservice. Like a raging forest fire that runs out of trees, the virus effectively limits its ability to spread by maiming or killing the host before he or she can transmit the virus to others. This may be the case with Ebola.

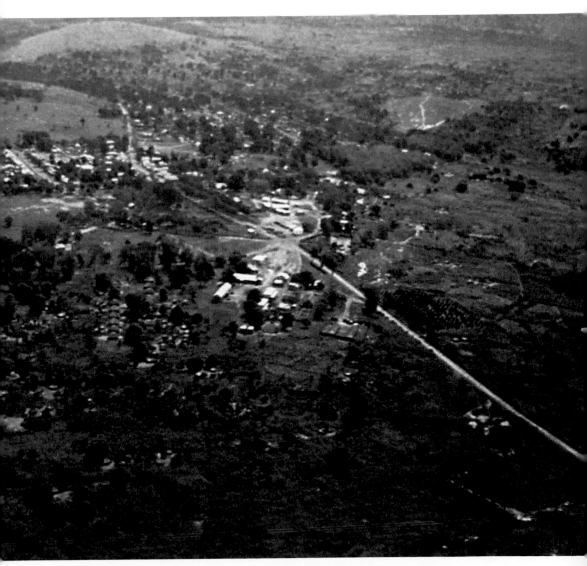

An aerial view shows the small village of Yambuku, Zaire, site of the deadly 1976 Ebola outbreak. The virus devastated the area within weeks. By quarantining the surrounding area, the virus was contained to Yambuku and western Sudan.

The best-case scenario for a virus is to keep its host alive as long as possible while replicating inside its cells. If it can do this without making the host so sick that he or she cannot go about normal activities, the virus has a greater likelihood of finding more hosts to infect and, therefore, greater opportunity to make more viruses. For example, the virus that causes the common cold generally makes its host feel slightly under the weather, but not ill enough to stay home from work or school or to cancel travel plans. This works as a benefit to the adenovirus, which now has an opportunity to spread far and wide, a chance it would not have if it killed rapidly or if the host was so ill that he or she stayed home and away from other vulnerable potential hosts.

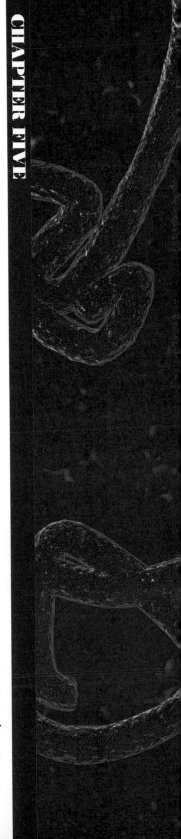

CHAPTER FIVE

THE IMPACT OF EBOLA

Though all epidemics disturb the economy of the affected geographic region to a certain degree, this is truer of some epidemics than others. Deadlier diseases have a greater likelihood of disrupting economic flow than milder ones, particularly in poor or very remote areas that are already cut off from larger trade routes and with few sources of income and few items to trade or sell. This is certainly the case in the areas of Yambuku, Nzara, and Bundibugyo, Uganda, where the most recent Ebola outbreak occurred. Cash crops in Yambuku include palm oil, rice, coffee, cocoa, and rubber. These items, as well as the meat and hides of hunted animals, are exported to surrounding areas in Sudan and Uganda in exchange for their goods, including cloth, metal utensils, and other desired items.

In addition to disrupting trade, the deaths caused by Ebola in these countries—when coupled with the impact of several other much more prevalent deadly illnesses endemic to these areas, such as HIV/AIDS, tuberculosis, and malaria—have reduced the national workforce and, therefore, productivity in the times of outbreak. This is particularly an issue with

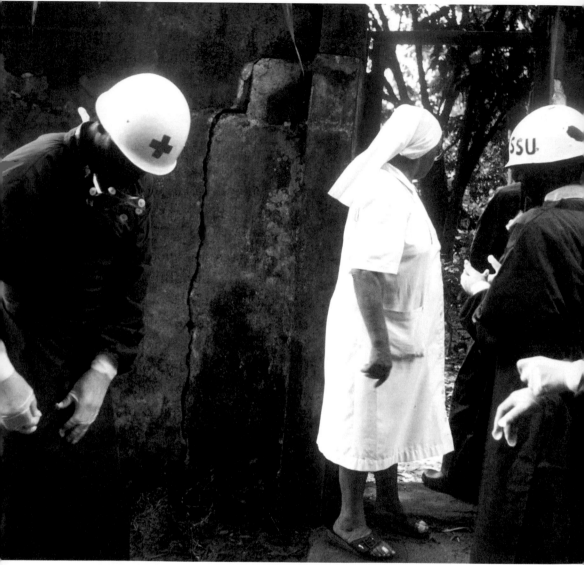

Health care workers in Kikwit, Zaire, disinfect town residents, local hospital workers, and buildings that may have been exposed to the Ebola virus during the 1995 outbreak.

regard to health care workers who are already in short supply. These individuals are at very high risk of contracting Ebola from their patients given the close contact they must maintain and the shortage of protective equipment, such as gloves,

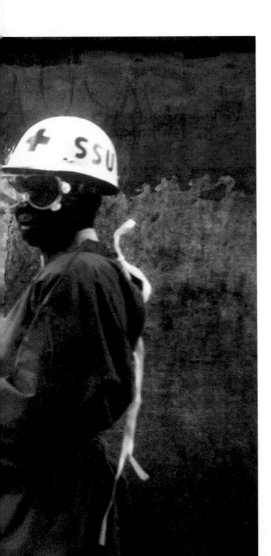

gowns, goggles, and other barriers. For example, by the end of the first Ebola outbreak at the Yambuku Mission Hospital, thirteen of seventeen medical workers had been infected with the Ebola virus. Eleven of them died. With so few medical staff, the hospital was forced to close. Also, Ebola scares in the affected nations have diminished an already low level of tourism to these areas, a frustrating fact given that many of these nations are struggling to increase the number of tourists in order to bring additional, much needed money to their economies. Should Ebola ever become as prevalent as HIV/AIDS, tuberculosis, or malaria, the economic effects on these already struggling communities would be devastating.

The Impact on Families

The impact of Ebola on individual families was equally devastating. From an economic standpoint, if a member of a household who worked fell ill or died, they would no longer be able to provide for his or her family. In many cases, these families had very little to begin with and starvation was a realistic

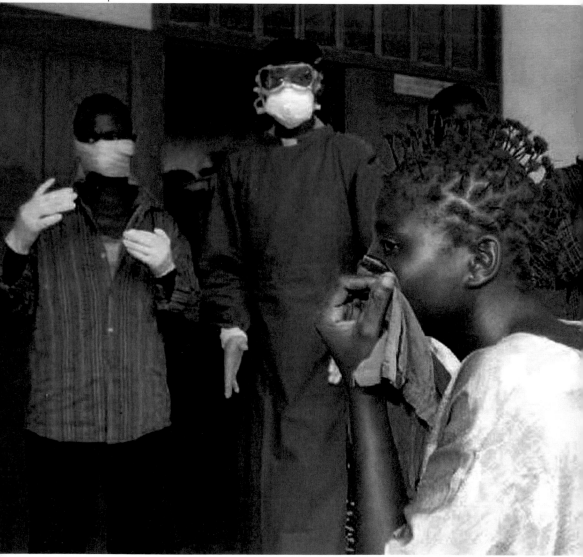

Family members of patients infected with Ebola eagerly await news of their loved ones' condition outside the Kikwit Hospital during the 1995 outbreak. Many of them may have been exposed to the illness in caring for or sharing living quarters or meals with the infected individuals.

possibility. The emotional impact of Ebola on a family likely caused even greater stress. Family members had to stand by as they watched their loved ones grow terribly ill and suffer terrible pain. They often watched them die. Worse yet, because

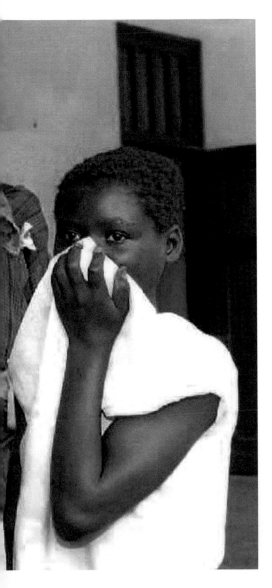

of the risk of contracting Ebola from their dying loved ones, family members had to make the difficult choice between protecting themselves and affectionately tending to a sick child, spouse, sibling, or parent. There was likely an issue of social isolation suffered by these individuals and their families as panic spread. Individuals thought to be ill were often prohibited from approaching healthy people, and their body secretions were avoided. They were often isolated to hospital units or, if none was available, to their homes.

The Social Impact

Funeral customs that involve important spiritual rites are also disturbed during outbreaks. In many of the Ebola-afflicted areas, funerals involve the preparing and washing of the body by family and friends. Often, food and excreta are removed from the body, which is then dressed and displayed publicly (laid out on a mat). The next day, the community gathers around the body, dancing and singing songs about the person who has died. The body is frequently hugged, kissed, and touched. Forbidding these rituals from taking place prevents the deceased individual's community from mourning properly. It makes the pain at the loss of a loved one worse, since his or her spirit cannot be sent properly from this world to the next. Anthropologists have been hard at work with epidemiologists

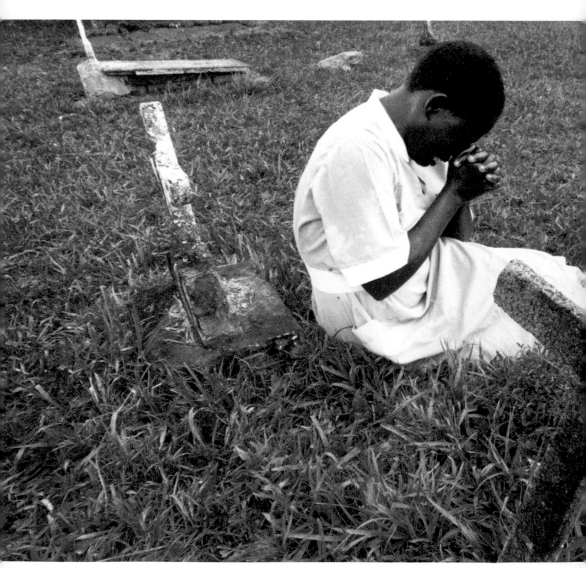

A Ugandan nurse breaks down in mourning after a coworker fell victim to Ebola after having treated several infected individuals. In many ways, these workers sacrificed their own health to provide care and comfort to their patients.

to help balance the need to respect these traditions while taking measures to prevent the spread of the Ebola virus.

Ebola greatly disturbed the balance of normal social relationships, as well as the relationships these communities

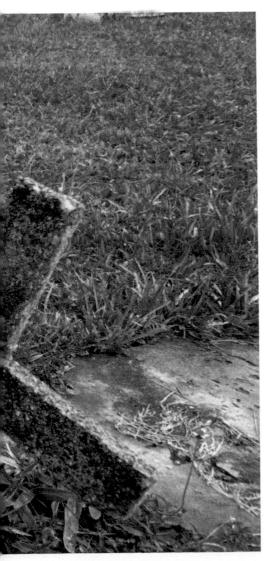

had with nature. Many individuals in the rural areas where Ebola has surfaced rely on animals from the surrounding jungle for their livelihood, dietary needs, and as part of long-standing social customs. Some coming-of-age rituals involve eating specific organs of animals, including hearts and livers, which are rich with blood. It is customary that carcasses are prepared in a particular manner by hand. Unfortunately, many of these customs are quite dangerous, since contact with animals carrying the Ebola virus is likely a primary route of infection. The government often bans the hunting and selling of wild game—particularly of chimpanzees and gorillas—and many long-standing traditions associated with it during outbreaks. The government has promoted the eating and selling of meat from domestic farm animals and fish, but such luxuries are usually in short supply or dependent on the season.

Ebola as a Weapon of War

The term "bioterrorism" refers to the use of a biological agent, such as a virus or bacterial strain, to cause death or disease in humans, animals, or plants. These agents can be spread via contamination of food and water, or by air. Very few agents are considered capable of causing a serious threat of widespread death and illness. Because it has no known treatment, a high death rate, and is easily spread among family members and others in close contact, Ebola is considered a Category A bioterrorism agent candidate, despite the fact that the virus is not spread via airborne transmission. In fact, some conspiracy theorists believe that the Ebola virus was man-made in a lab for the express purpose of using it as a weapon of war. Such theories have been disproved (and are unlikely). Though the risk of a bioterrorism event is generally very low, the consequences could be severe if one were to occur. As a result, the CDC and National Institutes of Health (NIH) have drafted guidelines that can be followed in the rare event of such an occurrence. Of course, should a vaccine or treatment become available, Ebola would likely be downgraded to a lower threat level.

While there is no guarantee that any of these worst-case scenarios will ever come to pass—in fact, the Ebola virus could disappear as quickly as it appeared—the world should be prepared. For that reason, health organizations, including the CDC, the NIH, the World Health Organization (WHO), and numerous smaller national and nonprofit research groups, have devoted resources, such as funding, researchers, equipment, and surveillance studies, in order to learn more about the Ebola virus and the illness it causes. They have called for studies to improve the detection of the virus, better recognition of symptoms of infection, faster transport of lab specimens for testing, better decontamination measures, and better means of containing the virus if it emerges again on a larger scale. Currently, all incidences of Ebola are carefully tracked, mapped, counted, and confirmed. On the whole, these groups have done a commendable job working together. Importantly, they also provide factual educational material to the public about Ebola and countless other health threats and do so in a manner that provokes reasonable concern without undue panic or alarm.

This raises an important issue that should be applied to the study of all emerging viruses and other health threats. In the age of the Internet, endless amounts of information about viruses, bacteria, medicines, bioterrorism, and scientific research are available to us. However, not all information is created equal. Much on the Internet, as well as in books and newspapers, is not quite factual. For this reason, it is very important that information about medicine and diseases be obtained from reputable sources. Many of these are listed at the back of this book. When it comes to emerging viruses like Ebola, it is crucial that information be factual so that sound decisions can be made. For the time being, Ebola seems to have receded back into the rainforests of Africa. Hopefully, it will remain there, but all it could take is one small exposure by an unsuspecting hunter, gather, traveler, or explorer to bring the Ebola virus out of its natural reservoir and into the human population.

The Global Impact

Needless to say, if the reach of the Ebola virus were to extend beyond the boundaries of the confined areas in which there have been outbreaks, or out of the tightly regulated labs in which the virus is housed and researched, there is a possibility for a pandemic outbreak. This would be particularly true if the Ebola virus mutates to a form that enables airborne transmission to other humans and if no vaccine or treatment is discovered. If Ebola infection via the airborne route becomes possible, it might only be a matter of hours before the population of the entire planet is at risk of exposure. If someone who unknowingly contracted the disease hopped on an international flight and coughed along the way, they would expose

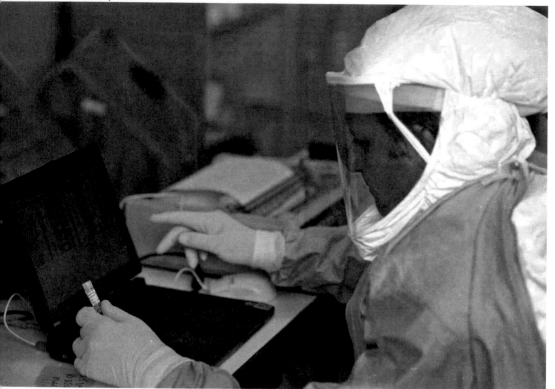

A CDC scientist wearing protective gear documents data collected after testing blood samples for the presence of Ebola at a Ugandan hospital in 2000.

all others onboard to the now contagious illness. On the other hand, should the virus mutate to an airborne strain in a quarantined lab facility for imported monkeys, human researchers who have thus far considered themselves safe might unknowingly bring the virus out of these protected labs and into the outside world. The scientists who first studied the Ebola virus knew from the outset that it could have this potential, though the likelihood of an Ebola pandemic currently is very slim.

TEN GREAT QUESTIONS
to ask a DOCTOR

1 Who is at risk for becoming ill with the Ebola virus?

2 What are the symptoms of Ebola?

3 Am I at risk of getting Ebola?

4 What kind of research has been done regarding cures and treatments for Ebola?

5 To which virus family does Ebola belong?

6 How many strains of Ebola are there?

7 Which Ebola strain has had the highest death rate?

8 What is an index case?

9 What do epidemiologists do?

10 What is the role of the Centers for Disease Control and Prevention in the United States?

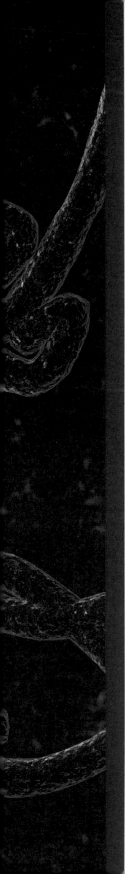

GLOSSARY

anemia A deficiency of red blood cells.

antibodies Proteins typically produced by the
immune system in response to the presence of
foreign substances (antigens), such as viruses or
bacteria. Antibodies aid in recognizing and fighting
infection.

antigen A foreign substance that produces an
immune response when introduced into the body.

antiserum Blood serum containing antibodies against
specific antigens that may be used to attempt to
transfer immunity to a disease to another individual.

biological warfare The use of bacteria, viruses, or
toxins to destroy humans, plants, animals, or food.

bioterrorism The use, or threatened use, of biological
agents to promote or spread fear or intimidation to
an individual, specific group, or population as a
whole for religious, political, ideological, financial,
or personal purposes.

DNA A molecule containing hereditary information
that codes for proteins. Genes and chromosomes
are composed of DNA. All living organisms contain
DNA, as do some viruses.

ecosystem A community of plants, animals, and micro-
organisms that, in combination with their physical
environment, functions as a unit. An ecosystem
can be as large as a rainforest and as small as a
rotting tree stump. If one element of an ecosystem
is disturbed or taken out of the equation, the rest
of the system becomes vulnerable to collapse.

electron microscope An instrument that uses
electrons, instead of light, to produce a magnified
image of an object up to two million times its
actual size.

emerging infectious disease A disease that suddenly infects new species or enters new geographical regions as a result of normal viral mutation or changes in human patterns of expansion or development.

endemic Prevalent in or peculiar to a particular locality, region, or people.

epidemic The occurrence of more cases of a disease than would be expected in a community or region during a given time period. A sudden, severe outbreak of a disease.

epidemiology The branch of public health dealing with the transmission and control of disease. The use of medical science and statistics to track population health and find causes of diseases in groups of people.

filovirus A virus that is a member of the family Filoviridae, or "the thread" viruses, like Ebola or Marburg. These viruses look like string or threads under an electron microscope.

hemorrhagic fever An illness caused by a viral infection and exhibiting fever and gastrointestinal symptoms, followed by destruction of blood vessels and a massive loss of blood.

host An organism in which a virus or other infectious agent can replicate.

immune response The body's defense against foreign objects or organisms, such as bacteria, viruses, or transplanted organs or tissue.

incubation period The time period between when a person is first infected with a disease-causing agent and the time when clinical manifestation of the disease occurs.

index case The earliest documented case of a disease that is included in an epidemiological study.

malaria A disease caused by a blood parasite spread by certain types of mosquitoes in tropical areas.

microbiology The branch of biology that studies micro-organisms, such as bacteria, viruses, fungi, and protozoa, and their effects on humans.

mutate To change the genetic material of an organism or infectious agent. This ability often allows a virus to change slightly over time and can make treatment more difficult or could expand the types of organisms it is able to infect.

nosocomial infections Infections accidentally acquired in a hospital during, and as a result of, medical care.

outbreak The sudden emergence of a particular disease.

pandemic An epidemic occurring over a very wide area, crossing international boundaries and usually affecting large numbers of people; a global disease epidemic.

Phase 1 clinical trial A highly regulated research project in which scientists test a new drug or treatment in a small group of people (twenty to eighty) for the first time to evaluate its safety, determine a safe dosage range, and identify side effects.

primate The highest order of mammals including humans, apes, and monkeys.

quarantine A period of isolation ordered to control the spread of infectious disease, particularly those for which there is no known cure or with a high mortality rate.

reservoir Any person, animal, arthropod, or part of the environment (soil or substance) in which an infective agent normally lives.

RNA A molecule similar to DNA, but usually single-stranded, containing information often used as a protein-building template.

supportive treatment Treatment given to prevent, control, or relieve complications and side effects of an illness and improve the patient's comfort and quality of life.

transmission Means by which infectious disease is spread to or among people.

vaccine A substance given orally or by injections that confers protection against a particular disease.

vector A carrier that transmits an infective agent from one host to another.

viremia A situation in which viruses enter the bloodstream, thus gaining access to all organs and tissues of the body.

virus A tiny infectious agent that is dependent on host cells for replication because they cannot reproduce on their own.

zoonotic An infectious disease that can be passed from vertebrate animals to humans.

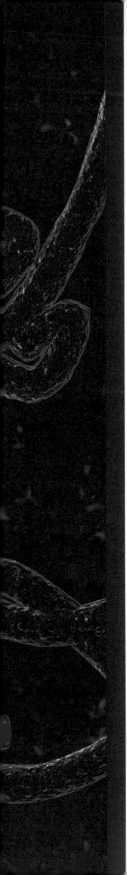

FOR MORE INFORMATION

Canadian Public Health Association
400 - 1565 Carling Avenue
Ottawa, ON K1Z 8R1
Canada
(613) 725-3769
Web site: http://www.cpha.ca
The Canadian Public Health Association is a national,
    independent, nonprofit, voluntary association
    representing public health in Canada with links to
    the international public health community.

Canadian Society for International Health
1 Nicholas Street
Suite 1105
Ottawa, ON K1N 7B7
Canada
(613) 241-5785
Web site: http://www.csih.org
The Canadian Society for International Health is a
    national nongovernmental organization that
    works domestically and internationally to reduce
    global health inequities and strengthen health
    systems.

**Centers for Disease Control
    and Prevention (CDC)**
1600 Clifton Road
Atlanta, GA 30333
(800) 232-4636
Web site: http://www.cdc.gov
The U.S. Centers for Disease Control and
    Prevention is a government agency at the fore-
    front of public health efforts to prevent and

control infectious and noninfectious diseases, injuries, workplace hazards, disabilities, and environmental health threats.

Clinical Trials

National Institutes of Health

9000 Rockville Pike

Bethesda, MD 20892

(301) 496-4000, TTY (301) 402-9612

Web site: http://clinicaltrials.gov

ClinicalTrials.gov offers up-to-date information for locating federally and privately supported clinical trials for a wide range of diseases and conditions. A clinical trial (also clinical research) is a research study in human volunteers to answer specific health questions.

Health Canada

Address Locator 0900C2

Ottawa, ON K1A 0K9

Canada

Web site: http://www.hc-sc.gc.ca

(866) 225-0709

Health Canada is the federal department responsible for helping Canadians maintain and improve their health, while respecting individual choices and circumstances.

HowStuffWorks

One Capital City Plaza

3350 Peachtree Road, Suite 1500

Atlanta, GA 30326

(404) 760-4729

Web site: http://videos.howstuffworks.com/sciencentral/2936-ebola-vaccine-video.htm

HowStuffWorks provides unbiased, easy-to-understand
explanations of how the world actually works, from car
engines to search engines, cell phones to stem cells, and
everything in between. The site is an online resource for
millions of people of all ages.

Mayo Clinic
Mayo Foundation for Medical Education and Research
200 First Street SW
Rochester, MN 55905
Web site: http://www.mayoclinic.com
A team of Web professionals and medical experts work side by
side to offer health information to help users assess symp-
toms, understand their diagnosis, and manage their health.

Merck Manuals Online Medical Library
One Merck Drive
P.O. Box 100
Whitehouse Station, NJ 08889
(888) 776-8364
Web site: http://www.merck.com/mmhe/index.html
The *Merck Manual of Medical Information–Home Edition*,
published through the Merck Pharmaceutical company,
translates complex medical information into plain language
for individuals interested in medical care who do not
have a medical degree.

National Institutes of Health
9000 Rockville Pike
Bethesda, MD 20892
(301) 496-4000
Web site: http://www.nih.gov/index.html
The National Institutes of Health, a part of the U.S.

Department of Health and Human Services, is the primary federal agency for conducting and supporting medical research.

National Library of Medicine/Medline Plus
8600 Rockville Pike
Bethesda, MD 20894
Web site: http://www.nlm.nih.gov
The National Library of Medicine in Bethesda, Maryland, is the world's largest medical library. The library collects materials and provides information and research services in all areas of biomedicine and health care.

World Health Organization
Avenue Appia 20
1211 Geneva 27
Switzerland
Telephone: + 41 22 791 21 11
Web site: http://www.who.int/en
The World Health Organization is a specialized agency of the United Nations that serves as a coordinating authority on international public health issues.

Web Sites

Due to the changing nature of Internet links, Rosen Publishing has developed an online list of Web sites related to the subject of this book. This site is updated regularly. Please use this link to access the list:

http://www.rosenlinks.com/epi/ebola

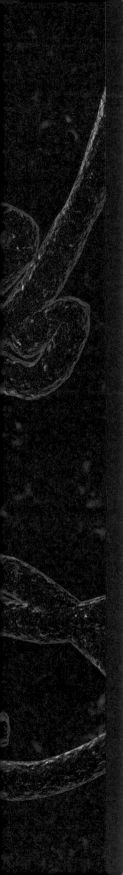

FOR FURTHER READING

Alter, Judy. *Vaccines*. Ann Arbor, MI: Cherry Lake
    Publishing, 2008.
Asher, Dana. *Epidemiologists: Life Tracking Deadly
    Diseases* (Extreme Careers). New York, NY: Rosen
    Publishing Group, 2002.
Friedlander, Mark P., Jr. *Outbreak: Disease Detectives
    at Work*. Minneapolis, MN: Twenty-First Century
    Books, 2009.
Goldsmith, Connie. *Invisible Invaders: Dangerous
    Infectious Diseases*. Minneapolis, MN: Twenty-First
    Century Books, 2006.
Heale, Jay. *Democratic Republic of the Congo*
    (Cultures of the World). Tarrytown, NY: Marshall
    Cavendish Children's Books, 2009.
Hodge, Russ. *Human Genetics* (Genetics and
    Evolution). New York, NY: Facts on File, 2010.
Peters, C. J. *Virus Hunter: Thirty Years of Battling Hot
    Viruses Around the World*. New York, NY: Anchor
    Press, 1998.
Pohl, Kathleen. *Looking at the Congo*. New York, NY:
    Gareth Stevens Publishing, 2008.
Raven, Peter H., Linda R. Berg, and David M.
    Hassenzahl. *Environment*. Hoboken, NJ:
    Wiley, 2006.
Royston, Angela. *Colds, the Flu, and Other Infections*
    (How's Your Health?). Mankato, MN: Smart Apple
    Media, 2008.
Ryabchikova, Elena. *Ebola and Marburg Viruses*.
    Aberdeen, MD: Battelle Press, 2002.
Sompayrac, Lauren. *How Pathogenic Viruses Work*.
    Sudbury, MA: Jones and Bartlett Publishers,
    Inc., 2002.

BIBLIOGRAPHY

Brooks, Geo. F, Butel, Janet S. and Morse, Stephen A. *Jawetz, Melnick, & Adelberg's Medical Microbiology*. 23rd ed. New York, NY: Lange Medical Books/McGraw-Hill Medical Publishing Division, 2004.

CBS News. "Experimental Ebola Vaccine Used on Human." 2009. Retrieved August 18, 2009 (http://www.cbsnews.com/stories/2009/03/27/health/main4897190.shtml).

Centers for Disease Control and Prevention. "Laboratory Biosafety Level Criteria." 2000. Retrieved August 14, 2009 (http://www.cdc.gov/OD/ohs/biosfty/bmbl4/bmbl4s3.htm).

Centers for Disease Control and Prevention Special Pathogens Branch. "Ebola Hemorrhagic Fever Information Packet." 2002. Retrieved July 29, 2009 (http://www.cdc.gov/ncidod/dvrd/spb/mnpages/dispages/Ebola.htm).

Garrett, Laurie. *The Coming Plague: Newly Emerging Diseases in a World Out of Balance*. New York, NY: Penguin Publishing, 1994.

Heymann, David L., ed. *Control of Communicable Diseases Manual*. 18th ed. Washington, DC: American Public Health Association, 2004.

Holmes, Bob. "Ebola Drug Found in Forest." *New Scientist*, 1999. Retrieved August 21, 2009 (http://www.newscientist.com/articlemg16321991.700-ebola-drug-found-in-forest.html).

McCormick, Joseph B., and Susan Fisher-Hock. *Virus Hunters of the CDC*. Atlanta, GA: Turner Publishing, Inc., 1996

National Institutes of Health. "Experimental Ebola Vaccine Trial." 2003. Retrieved August 16, 2009 (http://www.clinicaltrials.gov/ct2/show/NCT00072605?term=ebolaandrank=3).

Preston, Richard. *The Hot Zone: A Terrifying True Story*. New York, NY: Anchor Books,1995.

Villarreal, Luis. "Are Viruses Alive?" *Scientific American*, 2004. Retrieved August 16, 2009 (http://www.scientificamerican.com/article.cfm?id=are-viruses-alive).

World Health Organization. "Ebola Hemorrhagic Fever." 2008. Retrieved August 21, 2009 (http://www.who.int/csr/disease/ebola/en).

INDEX

A

airborne transmission, 7–8,
  16–17, 45, 62, 63, 64
anthropologists, 60
antibodies, 30, 40, 41, 43
antiserum, 30

B

Biocontainment and the
  environment, 48–54
Biosafety Level 1, 46
Biosafety Level 2, 46
Biosafety Level 3, 46, 48
Biosafety Level 4, 46–48
biosafety suits, 48
bioterrorism, 45, 62–63
bleeding out, 18–20
Bumba Zone, 13, 31, 49
burial and funeral customs,
  14, 26, 31, 59–60

C

Category A agent, 62
Centers for Disease Control
  and Prevention (CDC), 48,
  62, 65
coming-of-age rituals, 61
Congo rainforest, 21
Congo River, 21
conspiracy theories, 45, 62
crab-eating monkeys, 24,35

D

Decontamination showers, 48
DNA, 9, 49

E

Ebola-Bundibugyo, 25
Ebola–Ivory Coast, 24, 35
Ebola-Reston, 24, 35, 45
Ebola River, 6, 30
Ebola-Sudan, 24, 32–33
Ebola virus, the
  characteristics of, 7, 9–14
  containing, 48–54
  diagnosing, 36–38
  family impact of,
    57–59
  global impact of,
    63–64
  incubation period of,
    17–20
  myths and facts about , 45
  outbreaks of, 5–6, 13,
    22–24, 26, 29–34,
    48–51
  questions to ask a doctor
    about, 65
  research on, 11, 35,
    38–44, 62
  routes of infection, 14–17,
    21–22, 45, 63
  social impact of, 55–57,
    59–63
  symptoms of, 5–6,
    18–20, 22
  treating, 41
  types of, 24–26
  vaccine for, 40–44, 63
Ebola-Zaire, 22, 24, 25,
    29–31, 33
electron microscope, 7, 30
epidemiologists, 31, 60, 65

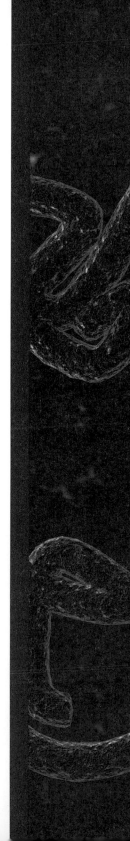

F

Filoviridae family, 10

G

Garcinia kola, 43–44

H

hemorrhagic fever, 6, 20, 30
HIV/AIDS, 6, 55, 57
host, 7–8, 9, 11, 49, 52, 53, 54

I

index case, 11, 13, 26, 33
Internet research on diseases, 63

L

light microscope, 7
Lyme disease, 11

M

Mabalo, Lokela, 13, 22, 24,
    26, 29
malaria, 18, 22, 55, 57
Marburg virus, 10, 30, 43
Mobutu, Sese Seko, 31,
    49–50
mutation, 14, 17, 26, 40, 63, 64

N

National Institutes of Health,
    44, 62
needles, 15, 22, 29–30, 52

Ngwete, Kikhela, 31
nosocomial infection, 15–16

P

pandemic, 4, 34,
    63–64
Phillipines, the, 24
Piot, Peter, 30, 48
polio, 38, 40

Q

quarantine, 31, 49–51, 64

R

replication, 9–10, 35,
    43, 52
reservoir, 11, 14, 35, 63
RNA, 9–10, 49

S

supportive treatment, 41
swine flu, 6, 15

T

tourism, 57
tuberculosis, 46, 55, 57

U

Uganda, 25
U.S. Army Medical Research
    Institute of Infectious
    Diseases, 43

V

vaccines, 38–44, 46, 52, 63
vector, 11
viremia, 15
"virus bomb," 15
viruses,
    best-case scenario for, 54
    characteristics of, 7–9, 14
    as living organisms, 49

W

World Health Organization, 62

Y

Yambuku Mission Hospital, 22, 26,
    30, 33, 34, 57

Z

zoonotic, 11

About the Author

Aubrey Stimola graduated from Bard College, where she majored in bioethics, an academic blend of biology and philosophy, two branches of study she feels are inseparable. She went on to work for a nonprofit public health organization in Manhattan, where she translated technical science and medical information into language comprehensible to a nonmedical audience. Her publications were designed to separate medical fact from fiction, the latter of which is abundant in the mainstream media and on the Internet. She performed a similar task for the New York State Department of Health before obtaining a master's degree in physician assistant sciences from Albany Medical College. Currently, Stimola practices emergency medicine in Saratoga Springs, New York, as a physician assistant. She continues to enjoy writing medical nonfiction for a broad audience.

Photo Credits

Cover (left), back cover (right), © www.istockphoto.com; cover (right), back cover (left) pp. 7, 21, 35, 46, 55, 66, 70, 74, 75, 77 © www.istockphoto.com/Monika Wisniewska; pp. 4–5 © Claude Mahoudeau.AFP/Getty Images; pp. 8–9, 10, 16–17, 23, 32–33, 37, 38–39, 46–47, 52–53 CDC; pp. 12–13 © Phillippe Psaila/Photo Researchers; pp. 18–19 © Pool/AFP/Getty Images; pp. 24–25 © Shinichi Murata/Photo Researchers; p. 34 © Carlos Palma/AFP/Getty Images; pp. 42–43 © Courtesy of USAMRIID Visual Information Service; p. 44 © Mark Noble/Visuals Unlimited; pp. 50–51 © AP Images; pp. 56–57 © Malcolm Linton/Liaison/Getty Images; pp. 58–59 © Christophe Simon/AFP/Getty Images; pp. 60–61 © Marcus Bleasdale-Telegraph UK/Zuna Press; p. 64 © Tyler Hicks/Getty Images.

Designer: Sam Zavieh; Editor: Nicholas Croce;
Photo Researcher: Marty Levick